Weight Loss In Theory and Practice

A Beginner's Guide to Intelligent and Permanent Weight Loss

RON KNESS

ISBN-13: 978-1546921844

ISBN-10: 1546921842

Contents

Disclaimer

This publication is for informational purposes only and is not intended as medical advice. Medical advice should always be obtained from a qualified medical professional for any health conditions or symptoms associated with them.
Every possible effort has been made in preparing and researching this material. We make no warranties with respect to the accuracy, applicability of its contents or any omissions.

See your healthcare professional before starting any diet, health or exercise program!

Assessing Your Current Health Situation

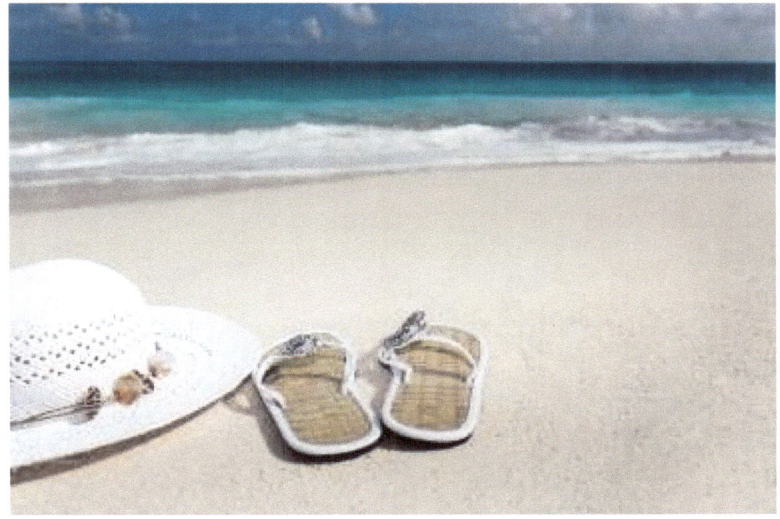

Losing weight is a journey. It doesn't happen overnight and you must be mentally and physically prepared in order to succeed in this journey.

The truth of the matter is that the majority of people can lose weight and keep it off if they follow the correct steps. In theory, the concept of weight loss is simple. You just need to expend more calories than you consume.

In practice, this may seem like a Herculean task and making the right changes can feel arduous and take a ton of self-discipline on your end. Like Jim Rohn once said, "Discipline is the bridge between goals and accomplishment." This is an undeniable truth as far as weight loss is concerned.

But here's the kicker... it doesn't have to be hard. In fact, weight loss is quite simple and straightforward if you do what's right in the right way and at the right time.

The first step will be to assess your current situation. You have to know where you are before you can get to where you want to get. You can't know where you're going if you don't know where you've been. It's crucial that you take a long and hard look at where you are in terms of your bodyweight and current fitness.

You'll need to do 4 things. Let's look at what they are.

Use the weighing scale

Get on a weighing scale and measure your weight in pounds or kilograms. While this is just a rough estimate of your bodyfat percentage, it will give you a general idea of how much you weigh.

Scale weight is not the be all and end all of tracking your weight loss. It can be deceptive and discouraging at times. You'll discover why in step 3 below.

Use a tape measure

Use a tape measure to measure the circumference of your bicep, waist, hips, chest, thighs and belly. Record the measurements so that you will have a future reference.

It doesn't matter whether you measure the left or right side of the body with the measuring tape. What really matters is that you always measure it at the same spots whenever you are tracking your weight loss progress.

Take a 'Before' photo

This is a very important step and with just about everyone having a smartphone, it just takes seconds to snap a photo of your body. Take one photo with you facing forward and one photo of your side profile... similar to what you see in the weight loss magazines.

Photos are probably the best indicator of how far you've come in your weight loss journey. A general rule of thumb is that in the first 30 days, you may see your weight drop a little and you'll notice the difference but your family and friends probably won't.

By the 60th day, there'll definitely be a visible difference and your family members will start to take notice that you are getting slimmer.

By the 90th day, just about everyone who knows you will have to admit that you've shed the pounds and you look fitter, healthier and have a certain glow about you.

The question now is... Will you reach day 90?

The photos that you take once every 3 weeks or monthly will keep you going. If you rely on the weight that you see on a scale, you may probably give up like thousands of people who do.

There's a reason for this. The scale does not show how much fat you've lost and how much muscle you've gained. People who start training after a long period of being sedentary can gain lean muscle quite quickly.

The body is craving muscle and grabs the chance to build some when you're eating and training right.

For example, if you lose 7 pounds of fat but gain 3 pounds of muscle at the end of a month, the scale will reflect a drop of only 4 pounds. This can be very discouraging to many people because they were expecting better results.

What they don't realize is that muscle is more dense than fat. So, by losing 7 pounds of fat, there will be a significant difference in your appearance.

Your jawline may become more pronounced. Your thighs may have stopped rubbing against each other when you walk and your arms may be much more toned.

But you can't see any of these results on a scale. That is exactly why you should take photos every now and then. When you compare your before and after photos, you'll be amazed at how much change there is... and these positive changes will spur you to do better and give more. You'll stay the course and be motivated to reach your weight loss goal.

See a doctor

This goes without saying. If you've health issues such as morbid obesity, blood pressure problems, etc. it's always best to consult a doctor first before embarking on any training program.

While you're at the doctor, you can also get your bodyfat percentage measured. This is probably the best gauge of how much fat you have and future visits will show how much you've lost.

The doctor may utilize calipers to determine this or he may use a fat loss monitor that uses bioelectrical impedance to determine your bodyfat percentage.

Whatever the case may be, you will have an accurate reading and an assessment from a qualified medical professional that you're good to go. If there are any precautionary measures that you should be aware of, your doctor will inform you about those.

This is about all you need to do to assess your current situation. In the next chapter, we'll look at the most crucial factor that determines if you'll lose weight successfully or join the majority of people who never succeed at it and battle with their weight all their lives.

You want to succeed, don't you?

Then read on...

Your Attitude Will Determine Your Altitude

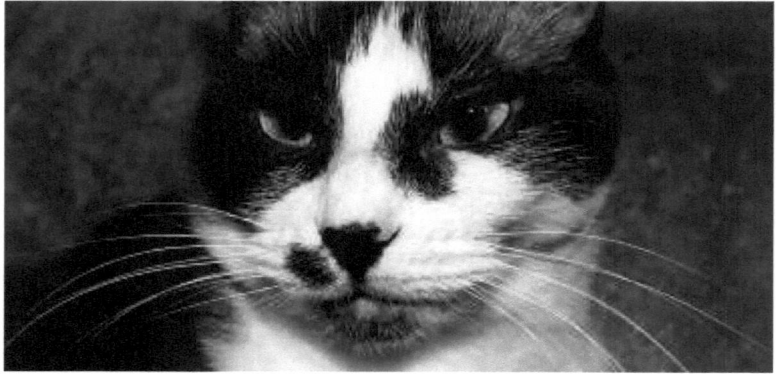

It may seem cheesy to read motivational lines when it comes to weight loss but there is a major mistake that most people make when it comes to weight loss. They assume that it's a physical thing.

They assume that they just need to eat right and exercise... and that's all they need to do. If that's the case, why then do most people fail to lose weight? Why is the New Year's weight loss resolution broken by over 90 percent of people?

The answer to this question must be seared into your mind and you must NEVER forget it.

"Weight loss is not a physical challenge. It's a mental one."

This truth is missed by most people. When you're on a diet and you know that you need to eat clean but you come across a glazed donut, do you steer clear of it or give in to temptation and chomp it down?

When you're supposed to workout, do you get up, get your gear and get the workout over and done with... or do you tell yourself, "I think I'll skip today and just do it tomorrow"?

Your success in your weight loss journey is the sum of small efforts repeated day in and day out. There will be days when the cravings for unhealthy foods are so strong that you feel depressed. There will be times when every bone in your body is groaning at the thought of the coming workout.

It's at times like these that your mental game must be on point. The only way to do this will be to define your why.

You're probably thinking, "Define my what?"

Not what... why. You must define your why. WHY are you trying to lose weight? What is the whole point to it all? Why don't you just want to stay overweight and obese?

The answers will vary... but no matter what your answer is, it will be based on an emotion. Most people do not want to lose weight just to be healthy. That's a boring thought that excites no one.

No no. People often want to lose weight and get fit so that they turn heads of members of the opposite sex. They want to be attractive. They want to be hot and sexy.

Or maybe it's a parent who wants to be around to see their children grow up. They know that if they allow their health to deteriorate, the consequences can be disastrous. This love for their children keeps them going.

Maybe the person has been diagnosed with a health condition that is so severe that they absolutely need to change their lifestyle or death is just around the corner. So they wake up and make massive changes to their lifestyle. This is a fear of death.

Almost all stories of successful weight loss are predicated by an emotion of some sort. THIS IS YOUR WHY... and you need to find out what your why is.

During those tough times when you're on the verge of giving up what you want most for what you want now, your 'why' will keep you going.

When you fall into a slump, your 'why' will give you the strength to push past the inertia and get the ball rolling. Your 'why' affects your attitude and puts the fire in your belly to keep going till you reach your weight loss goal.

Spend time thinking why you want to do want you want to do and WRITE IT DOWN. Make a few copies of what you've written and paste them all over the house... especially on the refrigerator door.

When you do this, you'll constantly be reminding yourself that there is a purpose for your weight loss and your purpose is greater than any temptation or challenge that life throws at you. With a mindset like this, success will definitely be yours.

Setting Goals and Meeting Them

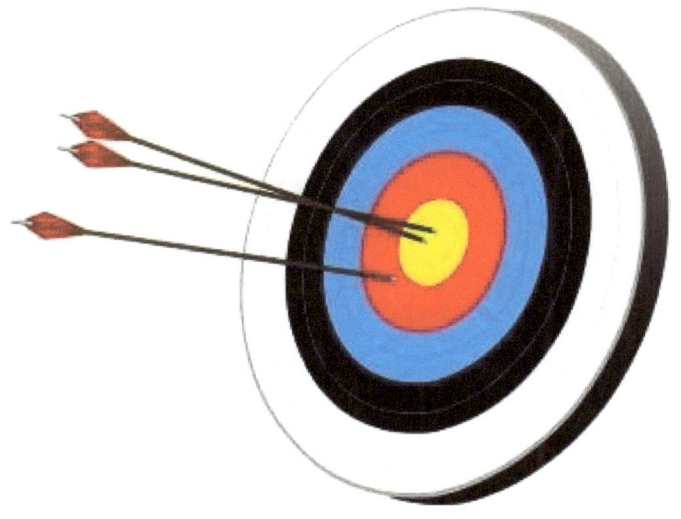

Here's the hard truth – the more overweight you are, the longer it's going to take you to reach your ideal weight. While this may seem like common sense, most people expect results overnight.

After 3 weeks of exercise, they expect to see all their excess weight gone and it really gets them down when they see nothing much has changed. They then throw in the towel because they feel like their efforts are not being rewarded.

Time for a reality check. Here are a few things you need to know.

- Losing 1 or 2 pounds of fat a week is normal.
  The more overweight you are, the more fat you will lose in the initial stages. As you progress, your weight loss results will start tapering down.

- There may be a week or two when the numbers on the scale just don't change... or might even go up a pound.

- Your caloric deficit is the most important factor.

- It takes time to lose weight.
  In order to set a weight loss goal, first you need to know what your ideal weight should be. You can calculate it using the link below.
  https://www.healthstatus.com/calculate/ideal-healthy-weight

Once you have a number, deduct it from your current weight. Let's assume you are 24 pounds overweight. We'll make a very conservative estimate of a 1 pound fat loss per week.

This means that you're looking at a 24-week stretch. That's about 6 months. Yes, you read that right. It may take you about 6 months to get to your ideal weight.

In all probability, you will get there sooner and it may take about 4 or 5 months depending on the aggressiveness as far as your dieting and training regimen. What you need to understand is that it will not take you 3 weeks or even 2 months to get to your ideal weight; the journey is much, much longer.

- You must understand that you gained the weight slowly and you will lose it slowly too. That's just the way things are and your body works at its own pace.

Do not try to do too much too soon. Many beginners make the mistake of training too hard and starving themselves to lose weight fast. What happens is that there may be an initial drop in weight by a few pounds and suddenly you can't lose any weight no matter what you do.

Your weight loss has hit a plateau because your body's self-preservation mechanism has been triggered. Your sudden reduction in caloric intake has set off an alarm within your body that makes it stubbornly cling on to its fat stores for future use.

This is how it protects you. To prevent this from happening, you'll need to gradually reduce your calorie intake.

Visit the link below and you'll see just how many calories you need to consume daily.
http://www.freedieting.com/tools/calorie_calculator.htm

Just by using this calculator and sticking to the numbers it gives you, your weight loss will be sure and steady. You'll always be at a caloric deficit and this is the biggest deciding factor when it comes to losing weight.

- You can exercise from morning till night and eat clean all the time... but if you are at a caloric surplus, you'll never see weight loss. **Remember this at all times**.

As far as setting goals go, now you know just how much weight you can lose and roughly how long it will take. So, you now can guesstimate a rough date that you can mark on your calendar. Set a date that states you will reach your ideal body weight.

Make small goals and meet them. Once you start cleaning up your diet and eating wholesome, nutritious food, your goal can be to slowly eliminate the detrimental foods out of your diet over time.

As far as your training regimen goes, your goal may be to get to the gym 3 or 4 times a week or walk daily. It doesn't have to be huge goals. Aim for ones that you can manage and each week, make small improvements.

In the next chapter we'll look at how you can change your life for the better with small baby steps.

Small Changes Make Big Differences

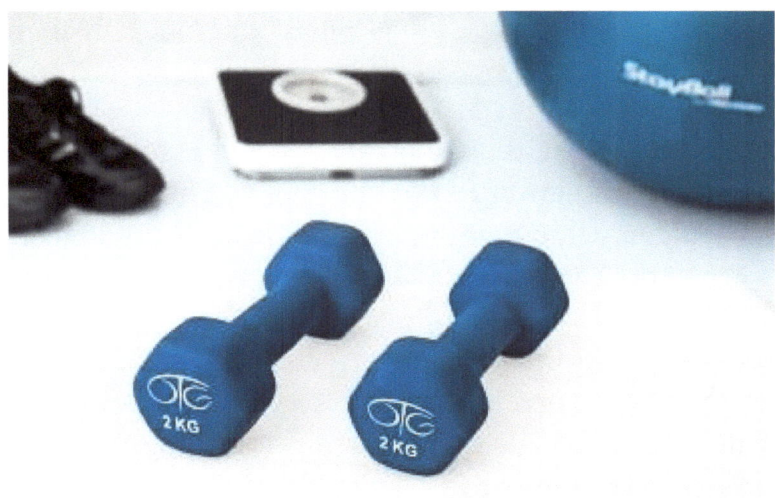

Small daily improvements are the key to staggering long-term results. This is a powerful truth that when applied to any part of your life will take you to new heights in personal achievement over time.

When you're trying to lose weight, at least 80 percent of your focus should be on your diet.

You absolutely cannot out-exercise a poor diet.

Eating habits are extremely difficult to break because the body responds very fast to any change in your diet. For example, if you eat sweet foods often, your body will develop a sugar addiction that you may not even be aware of.

If you suddenly try and remove all unhealthy and sweet foods from your diet, your body is not going to be pleased at all. You will develop sugar cravings, mood swings and may even feel sick. The body wants what the body wants. If you have ever tried to give up coffee, you know what I mean, headaches and all!

Some people try to give it all up at once and assume that they have enough will-power to stay the course. These same people suddenly find themselves binging in the middle of the night when their will-power has given out.

The only way to bring about lasting change is to introduce it gradually. Start a food journal and for the first week or so, write down every single thing that you consume. You'll then notice a pattern emerge.

Maybe you drink 3 sodas a day or have 2 bowls of ice-cream every night. Your goal now will be to make a small almost insignificant change that your body will barely notice.

For example, if you drink 3 cans of soda a day, drop it to 2 cans. You can do this for 2 weeks. Then drop it to one can and keep it like this for another 2 weeks... then maybe drop to half a can and finally none at all.

By doing this, you'll be gradually weaning your body off this unhealthy habit. Since it was done progressively, your body accepted the changes more readily. This is how you make small changes that lead to big differences.

The same applies to exercise. If you hate exercising, then do not immediately sign up for a gym membership that you'll never use.

Instead you may wish to go for a 10-minute brisk walk daily.

After a week, increase it to 15 or 20 minutes. Next, you may wish to throw in a few push-ups, sit-ups and squats after your walk. Don't push yourself too much. All you're trying to do is get your body used to the increased activity.

By doing a little each day, you'll be instilling a habit within you – the habit of daily or regular exercise. You can then start making small changes such as taking the stairs instead of the elevator or walking to the mall instead of taking the car or parking at the far end of the parking lot and walking in the rest of the way. If you take public transportation to work, get off a stop before or after your normal stop and walk in the rest of the way. These "tactics" make it easy to get in additional exercise without adding a lot of time to your day.

Every bit helps and contributes to your improvement. It may not seem like much but rest assured that when all these little changes are compounded over time, there will be a massive change in your results... and it will be for the best.

Inch by inch, life's a cinch. Yard by yard, life is hard.

Do not make the mistake that so many beginners make by trying to change their lives overnight. They clean up their diet so fast that all they ever think about is food. Or they workout so hard that all they ever think about is making excuses not to go to the gym and train.

Do not torture yourself. It may take longer to reach your goal but you will get there and when you do, you will have all the right habits in place to stay there.

Most people who do reach their weight loss goals often slide back to their old habits and gain all the weight they've lost – and more. Now they are worse off than when they started!

This is a proven fact. The reason for this is that they forced themselves to go all out and reach the goal as fast as they could... **but they never made the lifestyle changes a habit**. This is key, the changes you make have to be ones you can live with for the rest of your life.

A diet is something that will end and you'll go back to your previous style of eating; a lifestyle change is one that doesn't have an end and is something you will live with for the rest of your life.

By making small improvements, you'll be developing the right habits.

Motivation is what gets you started. Habit is what keeps you going.

Now keep going to the next chapter...

Understanding Nutrition and Applying It

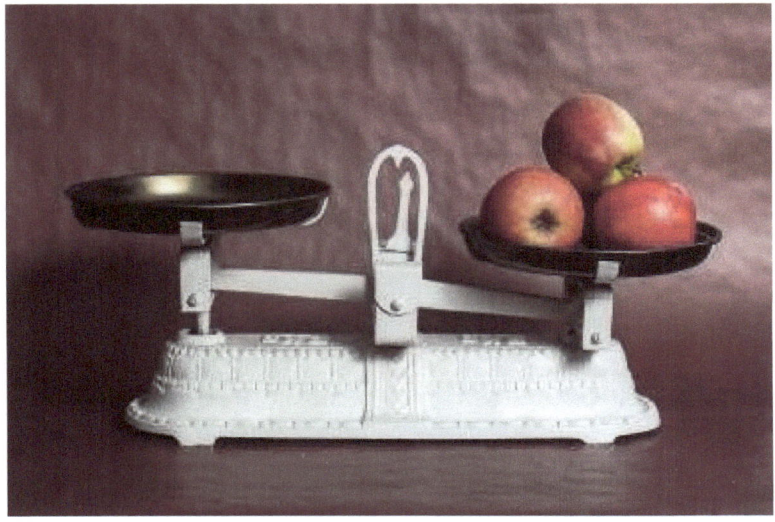

You may often have heard the terms 'micronutrients' and 'macronutrients' tossed around when reading about diets and nutrition. So what are they?

Micronutrients

Vitamins and minerals are just two examples of micronutrients the body needs. They are required in small amounts but play a crucial role in strengthening the body's immune system so that it can ward off diseases.

Macronutrients

Macronutrients are the substances that make up your foods. Your body uses them for energy, repair functions and growth.

Carbohydrates, proteins and fats are macronutrients. Your body absolutely needs all three types to function optimally. It is worth noting roughly how many calories the different types of macronutrients contain.

Carbohydrates - 4 calories per gram
Proteins - 4 calories per gram
Fats - 9 calories per gram

There are a few points worth noting.

You hold 3 grams of water for every gram of carbohydrate you consume. The more carbs you consume, the more water retention will occur in your body and you'll weigh more.

Most people become overweight or obese from overconsumption of carbs and NOT fat. In fact, one of the most effective diets on the planet is the ketogenic diet which involves minimal carb consumption with a focus on consuming fats and proteins. Very effective for weight loss.

You can lose weight by consuming junk food as long as you're at a caloric deficit. However, it's not healthy and the weight loss will be slower because it's not only about calories. The impact the food has on your body plays a role too.

Always combine a fat with a protein... or a carb with a protein. When you consume a food that contains protein, it is more metabolically expensive to digest this food. In other words, it takes more calories to break it down and digest it.

This is known as the 'Thermogenic effect of food'. Wikipedia defines it as '*the amount of energy expenditure above the resting metabolic rate due to the cost of processing food for use and storage.*'

Basically, what that means is that the body burns calories to digest proteins so it cancels out some of the calories in the food thereby reducing your chances of gaining weight. Some foods are known as negative foods meaning it takes more calories to digest them, than what they contain.

However, if you consume a fat and a carb at the same time, your blood sugar levels will spike and your body will release insulin because it is easier and faster to digest these macronutrients than protein. This will lead to rapid fat storage.

This is why foods such as donuts, fries, cookies, pancakes, chips, etc. should be avoided at all cost when you're trying to shed the fat. Or at the very least, they should be consumed minimally on your cheat days.

When trying to lose weight, your macronutrient ratios should be at 50% protein, 35% carbs and 15% fat.

Are you carb sensitive?

This is a HUGE problem that is the underlying cause for why fat people keep getting fatter... and the rate of weight gain is accelerated.

Some people are highly carb sensitive. When they consume even a little bit of carbs, they gain weight fast.

This is due to insulin insensitivity.

You're probably wondering what causes this. The answer is quite simple.

Let's assume you drink a can of sugary soda. The sugar in the soda will spike your blood sugar levels. Your body will release insulin to prevent your blood sugar level from getting too high (hyperglycemia).

Now if you were to drink 3 cans of soda a day, your body will keep releasing insulin to cope with these elevated sugar levels. Over time, your body will get desensitized to the insulin and your pancreas will have to keep releasing more insulin just to cope with the same amount of sugar.

When this happens, the excess insulin will be shuttled off to the body's fat stores through a chain of processes within the body. This will explain why overweight people often complain that they eat 1 slice of cake and gain 4 pounds.

While this is a bit of an exaggeration, you do get the point. A long time of consuming junk food and processed foods has affected their body's internal system.

Another very nasty consequence of insulin insensitivity is that it sets the stage for type 2 diabetes which is the leading cause of kidney failure, blindness and amputations. This is one of the worst diseases out there... and it all starts from a poor diet.

So what do I do if I'm insulin insensitive?

There are a few ways to reduce insulin insensitivity. Thousands of people will see rapid weight loss if they 'reset' their body's insulin sensitivity.

This is one of the biggest weight loss hurdles that most people aren't even aware of.

Fix your insulin insensitivity and it will become much easier to shed the stubborn pounds. Here are a few methods.

> ➢ Reduce your intake of all sugary and refined foods till you can eliminate them completely.

> ➢ Consume more foods which contain turmeric/ginger/garlic.

> ➢ Get enough sleep daily. This is very important. If you get insufficient sleep, consume some cinnamon. This will help attenuate the effects of the insulin resistance that arises from insufficient sleep.

> ➢ Lift weights.

> ➢ Run three times a week in a fasted state.

> ➢ Drink unsweetened green tea regularly. The gallic acid in the tea will improve your insulin sensitivity.

> ➢ Consume leafy greens and food rich in magnesium.

➢ Reduce or totally stop your intake of refined carbs like white rice, white bread, pasta, etc.

Just by following these steps, you'd have done the single biggest thing to help yourself progress faster in your weight loss journey. Get started on it today... and move on to the next chapter.

Popular Diets & Choosing One Which is Just Right for You

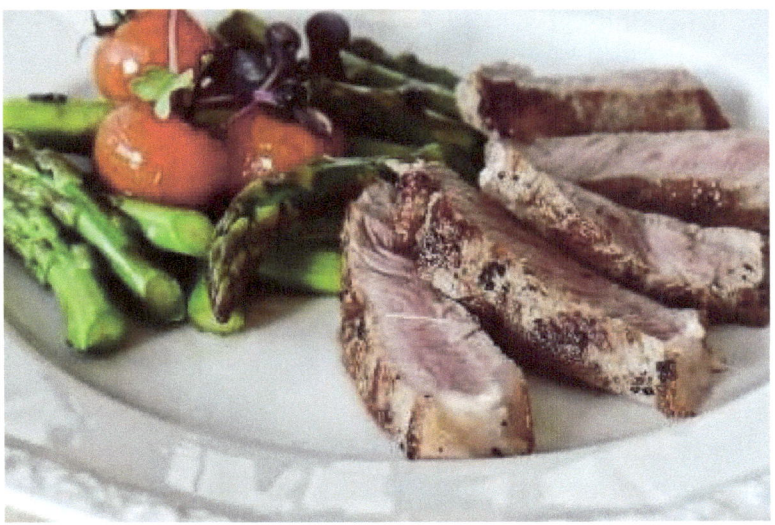

There are over 30 highly popular diets in the world. Just to name a few:

- DASH Diet
- MIND Diet
- TLC Diet
- The Fertility Diet
- Mayo Clinic Diet
- Mediterranean Diet
- Weight Watchers Diet
- The Flexitarian Diet
- Volumetrics Diet
- Jenny Craig Diet
- Biggest Loser Diet
- Ornish Diet
- The Traditional Asian Diet
- Vegetarian Diet

- Dr. Weil's Anti-Inflammatory Diet
- Slim-Fast Diet
- Spark Solution Diet
- Flat Belly Diet
- HMR Program
- Nutrisystem Diet

So which is the best one for you?

There is no right or wrong answer here because this book is not about teaching you to live your entire life on any one diet. While you may choose one to help you lose weight, ideally, the best thing that you can do is change your eating habits for the better.

A lot of diets have stringent rules and try to exclude certain foods that are deemed anathema to the diet. For example, the paleo diet doesn't allow you to consume artificial ingredients, grains and dairy.

This can be a nightmarish diet for people who love having the occasional cake and ice-cream. While there are paleo alternatives, they just don't quite cut it. Because of this, adhering to such strict diets can be a turn off for many people.

The key to succeeding with weight loss and keeping off the excess pounds is moderation. Life is too short for you to avoid the foods you love completely.

What you need to do is replace most of your unhealthy food choices with healthier ones... and occasionally indulge in the foods you love. Healthy eating should be a lifestyle choice and not because you're forcing yourself to be on a diet.

Include lots of vegetables in your diet. Have fruit for snacks. Replace sodas with water or unsweetened green tea. Cut down your intake of processed foods.

Follow the right macronutrient combinations. If your diet consisted mainly of single ingredient foods, you'd be just fine. A broccoli is a single ingredient food. Canned vegetable soup is not.

Like the late fitness guru Jack LaLanne once said, *"If man made it, don't eat it."*

As long as you are on track most of the time, it's fine to indulge in the occasional treat. Treating yourself (in moderation) to a food you love once every 4 or 5 days is just fine. In fact, it will give you a mental break and make you happier.

Drink lots of water because water helps in the fat loss process. Drink a glass of water before each meal. This will not only make you more full and prevent you from overeating, but it'll also keep you hydrated for your workouts.

Have a teaspoon of cumin seeds every day. This will help you lose 3 times more fat. It's such a simple practice but so powerful.

Consume one tablespoon of cold pressed coconut oil daily. This will further help in your weight loss progress. You must consume good fat in order to lose fat. When your body realizes that it has a steady supply of fat coming in, it will be much more ready to burn off its fat stores.

Coconut oil received a bad reputation in the past. However, recent studies have shown that it is one of the best foods around and prevents a myriad of health issues.

Carb cycling

This is another practice you may wish to adopt. Basically, you will consume minimal carbs for 3 to 5 days and will then have one cheat day where you consume carbs normally. This is a method used by fitness models all over the world to stay lean and ripped throughout the year.

Intermittent fasting

Another very powerful tool for burning up your fat stores. When you do intermittent fasting, you'll have an eating window and a fasting window. During the fasting window you'll consume no food but you can drink water.

Many people have a 16 hour fasting window and an 8 hour eating window. The shorter your eating window, the better. If you can have an eating window of 5 or 6 hours, you'll see the fat on your body melt off much faster since your body will burning it's fat stores for fuel most of the day.

Ultimately, your goal should be to be on an eating plan that you can maintain for as long as possible. You want to eat clean and healthy and at the same time, indulge in moderation.

Of course, you must be at a caloric deficit too until you reach your ideal weight.

Agonizing over stringent diets or giving up the foods you love is just going to be torturous and if you ever do cave in to temptations, you'll feel guilty. Once that happens, you may throw the diet out and start over-indulging in the foods you missed... and will end up back at square one.

Thousands of people go through this. But you won't because now you know better. You will aim for a sensible diet and moderation in all that you consume... and you will eagerly move on to the next chapter.

Introducing Exercise Into the Mix

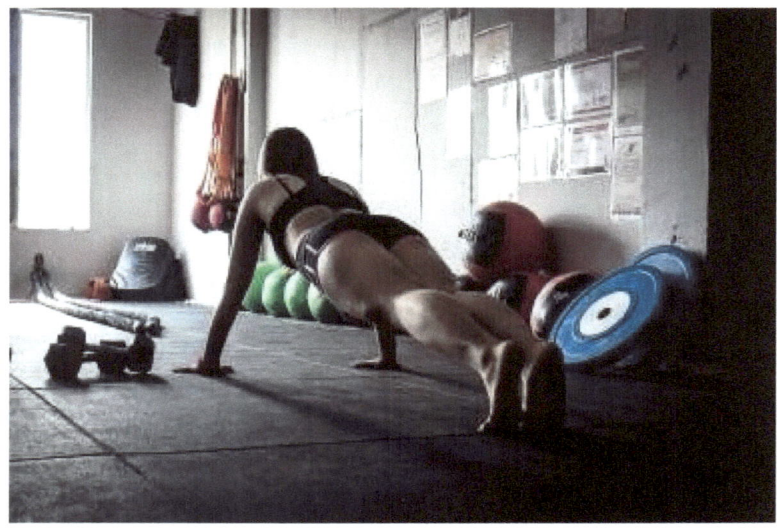

Surely you didn't think you'd be able to escape exercising, did you? ☺

While you can definitely lose weight through a caloric deficit alone, there are a few reasons why you should exercise too.

Firstly, it will speed up your fat loss journey. Regular exercise will boost your metabolic rate and put your body in fat burning mode. Not only will you be consuming fewer calories but you'll also be burning more calories. This winning combination will lead to faster fat loss.

Secondly, exercise tones your body. Losing weight through diet alone may make you slimmer but it will not make you look fit and lean. You can only do that with exercise. Only by training your muscles and stamina can you develop that lithe, toned body that turns heads.

Thirdly, regular exercise prevents cardiovascular disease and other health problems. Your body will get stronger and your immune system will be more capable of warding off diseases.

Exercise can be divided into 3 categories. Cardio, resistance training and stretching. All three are equally important and neglecting any one will be doing a disservice to your body.

Cardio

Most people dread cardio because it is exhausting. It is very common to see people pounding on the treadmills like hamsters on a wheel. The grim look on their face usually betrays how miserable they are. Exercise is torture for them instead of fun.

Running, swimming, cycling, rowing and many sports are cardio in nature. Pick one that you enjoy and go with it. There is no rule that says that you should only stick to running.

The goal here is to work your heart and break a sweat. You might as well have fun in the process. Another mistake that many people make is that they solely focus on cardio.

They may do 45-minute cardio sessions daily and expect to shed the pounds. This is usually counterproductive. When you engage in so much cardio, your body burns a lot of calories and it becomes very hungry.

So, it'll be very difficult for you to control your appetite when your body is craving for food. The best way to get around this will be to do about 20 to 30 minutes of cardio twice or three times a week. That's it.

As your stamina improves, you may wish to engage in short 15-minute high intensity interval training sessions (HIIT)… or even 4-minute Tabata protocol sessions. The intensity of these short workouts is so high that they'll actually burn more calories than the 45-minute steady state cardio workouts.

When a workout is high-intensity, your body goes into a state known as excess post-exercise oxygen consumption (EPOC). Your body will be in calorie burning mode for 8 to 12 hours after the workout is over.

You'll be burning a ton of calories. So, you've spent less time exercising but get more fat burning benefits. Your appetite will also not be raging because the workout session was short.

Resistance training
Resistance training can either be training with free weights or bodyweight training. This is a very crucial component of training and both men and women will benefit greatly from resistance training.

Contrary to popular belief, resistance training will not make a woman bulky. It takes a lot of work, weights, supplements and time to attain the physique of a bodybuilder. Most men struggle to gain mass. It's even tougher for women.

What resistance training will do is that it will give you a body that looks great in clothes and when not in clothes too. The curves in your body will be accentuated if you're a woman.

For men, the muscles will have definition and your body will have a solid, masculine form.

There are many other benefits of resistance training. We'll look at these in the next chapter.

Stretching
Almost everyone loses flexibility as they age. It would be a good idea to stretch for 15 to 20 minutes daily so that you stay limber well into your golden years. When you're flexible, you'll be less likely to get sprains and strains.

You may wish to join yoga or Pilates classes to become more limber and develop a stronger core.

Training in a fasted state

One highly effective technique to losing weight is to do a 20-minute cardio workout first thing in the morning. All you need to do is go for a 20-minute brisk walk on an empty stomach. That's it. There's no suffering involved here.

If you can't do 20 minutes, then aim for 15 or even 10 minutes. Over time, build it up to 20 minutes. When you walk in a fasted state, your body immediately burns its fat stores because your glycogen levels are low and it has no food to burn for fuel.

Over a period of time, these short 20-minute walks daily will burn a lot of fat. This is one of the easiest fat loss techniques you can use. Do not over-exert or do a high intensity session on an empty stomach. You want to be able to hold a conversation while you walk.

That's the kind of pace you should be at.

Steady state cardio Vs HIIT

Ultimately, most of your cardio workouts should be HIIT sessions. The days of long cardio workouts are long gone. They do more harm than good. Short 20 to 30 minute high-intensity sessions are far more beneficial and rewarding.

Furthermore, in our hectic society where time constraint is always a factor, these short workouts are a boon to the busy person.

It will take you a while to build your stamina to reach the level where you can do HIIT workouts. So, go slow and aim for slow improvements over time.

Always aim to beat your personal bests even if it's just a miniscule improvement. Finally, you will reach a point where you're fit enough for HIIT.

How many times a week to exercise?

Ideally, when you're trying to lose weight, you should aim for 5 to 6 days. Three days of cardio and 3 days of resistance training.

If that's too much for you, then 5 days will do too. Three days of resistance training and 2 days of cardio.

Alternate your workouts and you may wish to take a break every 2 days or every 5-6 days. Do what suits you and makes you feel comfortable.

The goal here is to get more active and move more than you're used to moving.

What if you don't feel like exercising?

This is a very normal feeling and even people who are gym rats feel like skipping workouts every now and then. The challenge is all the more difficult with the normal person.

If you feel like skipping a workout, don't do it. Tell yourself that you'll do just 10 minutes. That's all you need to do. Or even 5 minutes will do. You'll be surprised to see that once you start on the 5 minutes, you'll complete the 20 or 30 minute workout.

It's the inertia and old habits that are holding you back. You absolutely have to overcome those. Always remember, you just need to do 5 minutes... and see where you go from there. Anybody can do 5 minutes.

If you dread exercise all the time, your workouts are probably too difficult or you don't enjoy what you're doing. Tone down your workouts or find new sports or physical activities that you enjoy.

The guy who hates running may love swimming. The lady who abhors weight training may love rock climbing which is a form of resistance training too.

Find out what interests you and do it. All that matters is that you move more.

Is the gym too far?

In some cases, the gym may be too far from you. Just getting ready and going there and coming back can be a chore in itself. In cases like these, you're better off working out at home.

Get a set of DVDs such as P90X or Insanity Max and workout at home. You can do a ton of bodyweight training exercises at home or near a kid's playground that has pull-up bars, etc. You could even mount your own pull-up bar on your door frame. Make things as easy for you to workout.

Developing the habit of daily exercise is difficult as it is. Do whatever you can to ease the process.

Dealing with muscular aches

The only time you may give yourself a break from exercise is if you have muscular aches all over your body. This can happen when you're new to exercise and it invariably happens to all of us who've led sedentary lives for a while.

The lactic acid released by the muscles is causing the pain. You can either allow yourself an extra day or two to rest or alternatively, you may wish to do some light exercise such as going for a walk or a leisurely bike ride. This will help burn a few calories.

In some cases, if your biceps and upper body aches, you can always train your leg muscles.

Stay focused and exercise regularly. You must be stronger than your excuses and it's when you feel like skipping your training the most that you absolutely must get up and do that 5 minutes. This will boost your self-esteem and you'll develop the mindset of a winner.

And you're a winner, aren't you? Of course you are! You're still reading this... and you should carry on reading the next chapter.

The Importance of Resistance Training

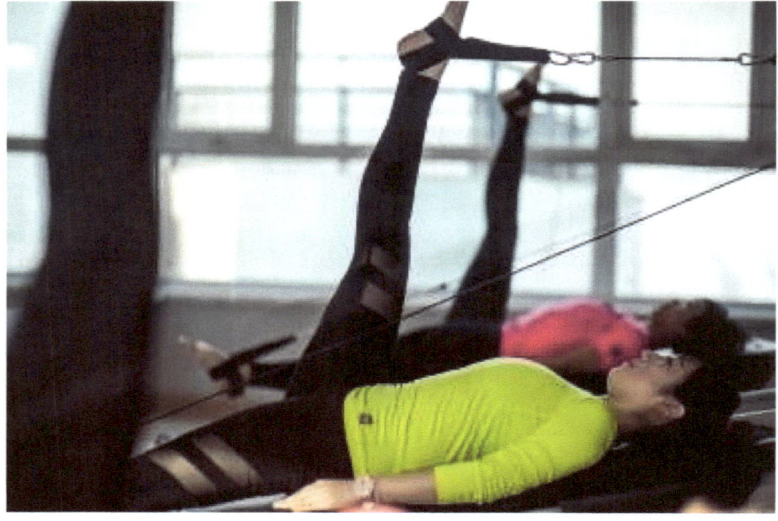

It was mentioned in the earlier chapter that resistance training is one of the key components of a well-balanced training program. Examples of resistance training are bodyweight training and training with free weights.

Many of the cool, sleek looking machines that you see in gyms are usually created for resistance training. They're designed to target specific body parts. While they do serve a purpose, you're better off sticking to free weights.

Now let's look at a few reasons why resistance training is so beneficial to you.

It boosts your metabolism

When you lift heavy weights, your body exerts and the muscles get a hard workout. When you're trying to lose weight, your resistance training should mostly comprise of full-body workouts.

Unlike bodybuilders who train one or two body parts a day, you should be doing several different exercises that target muscles all over the body. A sample workout would be like the one below.

Sample circuit – Do 2X or 3X per workout

- Deadlifts – 45 seconds followed by 15 seconds rest
- Push-ups – 45 seconds followed by 15 seconds rest
- Squats - 45 seconds followed by 15 seconds rest
- Hanging leg raises - 45 seconds followed by 15 seconds rest
- Burpees - 45 seconds followed by 15 seconds rest
- Lunges - 45 seconds followed by 15 seconds rest

By doing the workout above, not only would you have targeted several different muscles in the body but the minimal rest would have made the resistance training workout take on a cardio nature.

So, you'll be toning your muscles and improving your stamina at the same time. You'll be killing two birds with one stone. Not only that, but the workout will be exhausting and put you in calorie burning mode for several hours after your training session is over.

This will help you burn more calories overall and lose weight faster than you ever expected.

Lose 30 to 40 percent more fat
Studies have shown that resistance training helps you burn more fat. Point 1 explained why. What you need to do is incorporate resistance training in your workout to tap into their effectiveness at shredding the excess fat of your body.

More muscle = More calories burned at rest
Muscles are metabolically expensive to maintain and your body burns more calories when it's at rest if you are muscular. That's why you may notice that muscular people eat more and still stay lean… while those who are fat just get fatter.

It's the muscle mass at work here. The more muscle you build, the more calories you'll burn even if you're not working out. At this rate, you'll reach your weight loss goal quickly and you'll look really good when you do.

Better body tone
When you lose the excess fat and get more vascular, your muscles will look more defined and have a '3D effect'. If you looked at the weight of bodybuilders, you'll be amazed to see that despite looking massive, they're really not that heavy.

This is because muscle is denser than fat and takes up less space. Since they're lean, their muscles look more pronounced and give the impression that they are bigger than they really are.

While you may not wish to have the appearance of a bodybuilder, when you do resistance training and lose the fat, you'll look really good.

It takes ages to develop the physique of a bodybuilder and most of them are on muscle enhancing substances.

To someone like you who is trying to lose weight, this is a non-issue. All you'll see is a leaner, well-toned body like what Bruce Lee had... or if you're a woman, then you'll be fit and sexy like Jessica Biel.

Live longer

It's been proven that people who engage in resistance training regularly all through their lives, age better and stay fitter. If you look at the actor, Sylvester Stallone, you'll see that he is over 70 and still in excellent shape. This is a result of years of resistance training.

The same applies to other movie stars like Dolph Lundgren, Van Damme and Arnold Schwarzenegger. Despite being older, they still have muscles bigger than most guys half their age have.

This is the beauty of resistance training. It will serve you well in your later years and keep you tough and rugged while your peers will be limping around gingerly because their body is weak due to a lifetime of neglect.

Develop stronger bones

Another benefit of resistance training is that it will develop stronger bones in your body. Your tendons and ligaments will also get stronger.

Bodyweight training VS Free weights

If you prefer not to train with weights and keep things 'natural' there are a ton of bodyweight training exercises that are just as challenging. In fact, certain bodyweight exercises are so difficult that even people who have been training with free weights for years can't do them.

Planche pushups, front levers, V-sits, pistol squats, etc. are some of the most difficult bodyweight exercises in existence. If you can do them, you can rest assured that you will be strong and lean.

There are hundreds of bodyweight exercises and variations that will keep you busy for a long time. By the time you master them, you'd have reached your weight loss goal and be hard as nails.

It's next to impossible to get bulky with bodyweight training. So, if that's a concern of yours, bodyweight training has your name written all over it.

To see a variety of bodyweight exercises, all you need to do is go on YouTube and search for these exercises and try them out. Always be safe and approach the training in a sensible manner.

It would be good to mix bodyweight training with free weights. Neither is better than the other.

The goal here is to work your muscles and it doesn't matter which method you choose as long as you get there.

Many people feel intimidated going to a gym and would prefer to train at home. Others find it a hassle and some even balk at the cost of the gym memberships.

Some folks are even put off at having to use machines that have other people's sweat on them

The good news is that your muscles do not care where you work out. So you can either get free weights and train at home or just do bodyweight training in the privacy of your own home. Just make sure resistance training is part of your workout regimen.

Smartphone Apps & Wearable Devices to Enhance Weight Loss

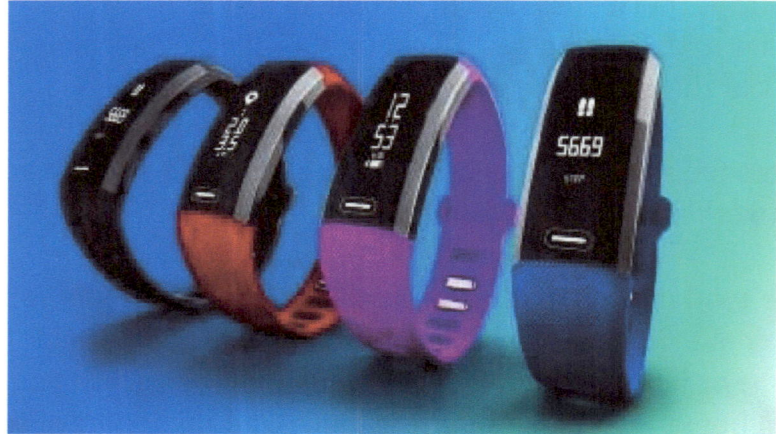

Do you need smartphone apps and wearable devices to lose weight? The answer is no... and the next question is, "Do they help?"

This time the answer is yes. While the apps and wearable devices do not guarantee weight loss, they make the journey more fun and slightly easier. We'll look at a few popular apps and wearable devices and you can decide if your need them.

Weight loss apps

Lose It

This is a free app that will help you create a weight loss plan that is suitable for you. It has a built-in food database to track your calories so that you can stay at a caloric deficit. It also has options that allow you to sync it with other fitness apps so that tracking your fitness becomes a breeze.

My Fitness Pal

This is another highly popular app created by the Under Armor brand that is all the rage these days. You can use this app to track your food intake and sync it with apps like Fitbit and Runtastic.

7-Minute Workout App

This is a fantastic app that will help you get a quick 7-minute workout if you're short of time. This is a typical example of a high intensity workout where you have a series of exercises that are executed quickly. You'll get your heart pumping and your calories burning with this app.

Click here to use 7-Minute Workout App

Wearable devices

Fitbit Charge 2

This device will help you track the number of steps you've taken daily and also your heart rate. The current goal these days is to get at least 10,000 steps a day.

While you shouldn't obsess over this number, it doesn't hurt to hit the quota on days when you're not training. The heart rate monitor will also help you know if you're training at your VO2 max.

Sony 4GB Sports Wearable MP3 Player

There's nothing like good music to motivate you while you work out. You can find a wide variety of MP3 players that you can wear during sports activities.

Unlike conventional mp3 players that have wires from the earphones, with these wearable devices you will not need to worry about dangling wires.

You have freedom of movement and also heart thumping, exciting music to keep you going and giving your best during your workouts.

Ankle weights

Bet you didn't see this one coming. It's old school and it's almost zero tech but it sure is useful. Just strap on the ankle weights when you're running or stair climbing or even walking. Every step has added resistance and you'll be burning more calories.

Even resistance training becomes more difficult when you have these on. Pull-ups, burpees, tuck jumps, hanging leg raises and many other exercises increase in difficulty when you've got ankle weights on. Even more, try using wrist weights at the same time. Just don't overdue it!

The more effort you expend, the more calories you burn. The more calories you burn, the more fat you lose. It's that simple. Ankle weights are inexpensive and definitely the first wearable 'device' you should get... even if they don't seem like much fun.

Making Diet & Exercise a Lifestyle Choice

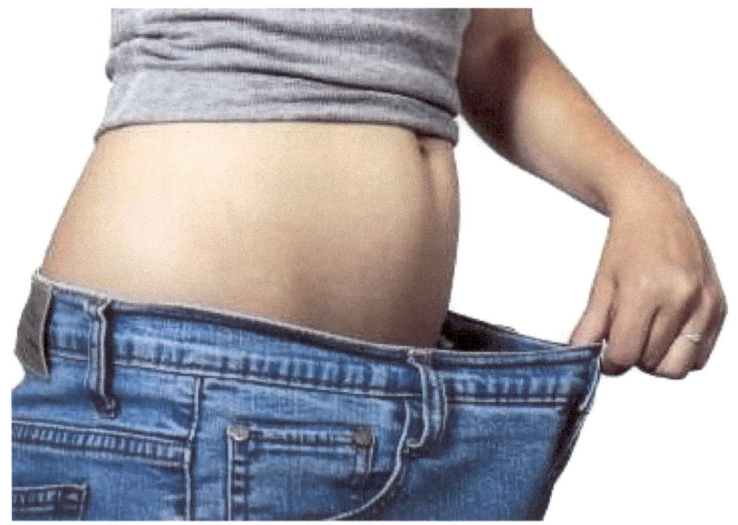

Congrats on making it to the end of this book. The hard truth is that the majority of people who started on this guide would have stopped reading halfway... just like how most of them will give up on their weight loss journey and never see their dream body materialize.

This is an uphill journey and you must have determination, dedication, and the three P's - persistence, perseverance and patience - to get to your destination. It can be done... but it will take a while.

And once you get the body you desire, it will be of paramount importance that you maintain the good habits such as healthy eating and regular exercise to keep the excess pounds from creeping back on. Once in maintenance mode, just add in a few calories to keep your weight around goal. Keep your exercise level the same.

Once you have the right lifestyle, staying fit, lean and healthy will be a breeze. Always focus on developing the right habits. If you're in control of your habits, you're in control of your life.

Coming to the end of this book is just the first step. You'll need to apply whatever you've learned and keep going even when the results that you're hoping for are slow to come.

It will be easy to lose steam when you're forging ahead. There will be times when it will seem like too much effort. Always look at your 'why' and realign yourself.

There are a list of quotes below that you may wish to print out and read whenever you feel like you just can't keep going anymore. Refer to them and read and re-read them till they soak into your spirit and refresh you.

- Blood, sweat and respect. The first two you give. The last you earn. Give it. Earn it.
- Dead last finish is greater than did not finish, which trumps did not start.
- Discipline is just choosing between what you want now and what you want most.
- Excuses burn zero calories.
- If it doesn't challenge you, it doesn't change you.
- If it was easy, everyone would be doing it.
- If it's important to you, you'll find a way. If it's not, you'll find an excuse.
- If you eat what you have always eaten, you'll weigh what you have always weighed.
- If you're tired of starting over, stop giving up.

- In life you have 3 choices. Give up, give in or give it your all.
- Life never gets easier. You just get stronger.
- No rest is worth anything except the rest that is earned.
- Nothing tastes as good as being fit feels.
- Nothing will work unless you do.
- Pain is temporary. Quitting is forever.
- Sacrifice is giving up on something good for something better.
- Suck it up... and one day you won't have to suck it in.
- Suffer the pain of discipline or suffer the pain of regret.
- Sweat is fat crying.
- The only bad workout is the one that didn't happen.
- What you eat in private eventually is what you wear in public.

When you feel like quitting, think about why you started. You don't have to be great to start... But you have to start to be great.

All the best in your weight loss journey and if you follow the advice in this guide and stay the course, success is inevitable. Difficult roads often lead to beautiful destinations. Yours is waiting for you.

Other Relevant Books by This Author

If you would like to read more relevant books about this topic, here is a list of the CreateSpace links, titles and descriptions from this author:

https://www.createspace.com/6131862

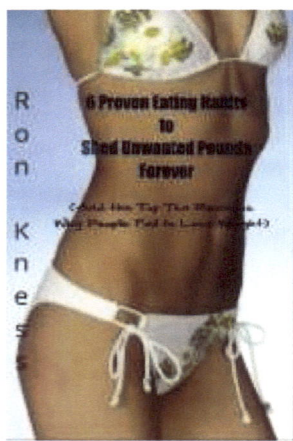

6 Proven Eating Habits to Shed Unwanted Pounds Forever: (And the Top Ten Reasons Why People Fail to Lose Weight)

One reason most people fall off the weight loss wagon after making heart-felt and sincere commitments is that the new habits they're trying to form are stressful and set up to make them fail.

But my book - "6 Proven Eating Habits to Shed Unwanted Pounds Forever" - is different; it charts a weight loss plan that can help you make lifetime changes that will help you maintain your ideal weight. It's the little habits which can make a huge difference and the advice contained in this book will be both obvious and eye opening.

Within these pages, you'll learn how distractions can cause mindless eating and pack on the calories without you even realizing it. Portion control is also a big factor in achieving your weight loss goals – even the celebrities lose unwanted pounds by watching their portions.

And finally, learn how to make smart choices when eating out.

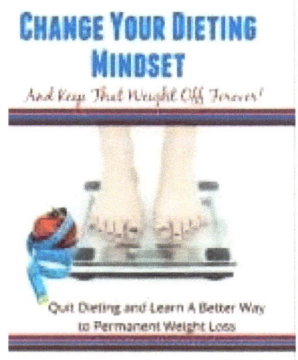

Change Your Dieting Mindset and Keep That Weight Off Forever: Quit Dieting and Learn a Better Way to Permanent Weight Loss

Change the way you view "dieting" and never suffer the frustration of yo-yo dieting and weight gain again.

What is the answer to permanent weight loss?

Simple. You need to forget all the incorrect weight loss information you have been given, get off the "diet merry-go round" and learn the healthy weight maintenance formula that will bring permanent and lasting results!

This information works for men or women. And it doesn't matter how young or old you are.

It works even if you have tried to lose weight in the past, and failed. It works and works well because…

It is NOT temporary
It is NOT restrictive
It is NOT depriving
And it is NOT another "diet"

When you understand the correct formula and what components make up that equation, healthy weight management is within your reach and that is exactly what you get with "Change Your Diet Mindset and Lose Tat Weight Forever".

Get your copy now and stop losing that same 20 pounds over and over!

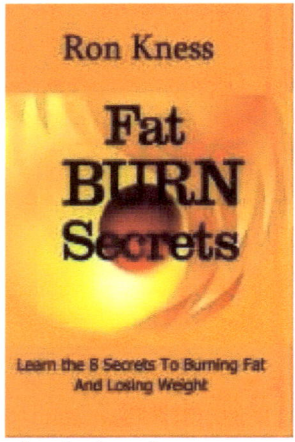

Fat Burn Secrets: Learn the 8 Secrets to Burning Fat and Losing Weight

Now you don't have to blindly spend hours of vigorous training and exercise in the gym anymore.

With this blue print for all exercisers out there, you will discover the importance of this amazing combination: making smart food choices in your daily lifestyle and choosing the right work out for your physical endurance.

Follow the easily learnable techniques in Fat Burn Secrets to obtain optimal results and strip that ugly fat off your body, once and for all.

Topics that Fat Burn Secrets covers include:

- Discover the differences between good fats and bad fats. Learn which unhealthy foods with bad fat that you should avoid and strategize a weight loss diet to lose those extra pounds

- Get fit and healthy with the right mindset. Achieving your ideal body shape takes more than just regular exercise and healthy eating. You need to develop a positive and motivated mind set to keep yourself going

- Find out the ninja secrets behind the slim figure of celebrities and apply the successful methods practiced by them to achieve the body that you've always wanted

- Choose the right cardio workout that suits the physical endurance of your body. Combine low intensity and high intensity cardio workout to strip that fat off your body faster

- Lose weight the right way to avoid the yo-yo effect. Be aware of the causes that can lead to this effect so that you won't regain all the fat that you've previously lost

- Practice yoga as a gentle form of exercise and stress management. If you're a beginner and don't know where to start… Perfect. You can learn all the basics with these easy and relaxing poses

- More fat-inducing foods that you should avoid on a regular basis. Fat Burn Secrets will reveal to you why food flavoring like corn syrup and MSG is hazardous to your health

- Are diet supplements recommended for you? Should you take them? Instead of regularly consuming them, why not try out some alternative ways to eating healthier to ensure your body absorbs all the nutrients that it needs

- Detoxification is now becoming a popular trend among dieters to ultimately burn those excess fats. Learn a variety of detox drinks that will surely give your system a good cleanse like never before

- Getting rid of "Love Handles" has always been a challenging feat. But fret not, because with Fat Burn Secrets' step-by-step exercises, you'll be getting rid of these stubborn fats in no time

- And much more to be uncovered in this fantastic game plan!

To sum it up, you'll learn how to:
- Start feeling energetic and be ready to take on the world!

- Crank your metabolic rate up a few notches

- Burn body fat the right way to reveal toned-looking physique hidden beneath layers of unwanted fat

- Get incredibly shapely hips and thighs and lean, toned abs

Get your copy today; start burning fat tomorrow!

About the Author

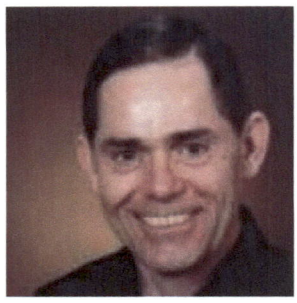

I have published over 125 books on Amazon for Kindle, CreateSpace and other publishing platforms.

While most of my books are on health and fitness in general, as I age (now 65) at the time of this writing) my topics of interest are geared toward aging baby boomers and older.

Besides my own writing, I also ghostwrite ebooks, books, reports, articles, blogs and do Kindle conversions for clients on a variety of topics.

Today my wife and I are retired from our careers and live in Gold Canyon, AZ. I now write as a retirement business where you'll find me happily sitting in my office typing away on my laptop as I work on my next book or ghostwriting project . . . that is if we are not traveling on a cruise ship - our new-found mode of travel.

www.ingramcontent.com/pod-product-compliance
Lightning Source LLC
Chambersburg PA
CBHW050825290526
45792CB00001B/263